THE

FATTY LIVER

DIET

COOKBOOK

SARAH JACK

1

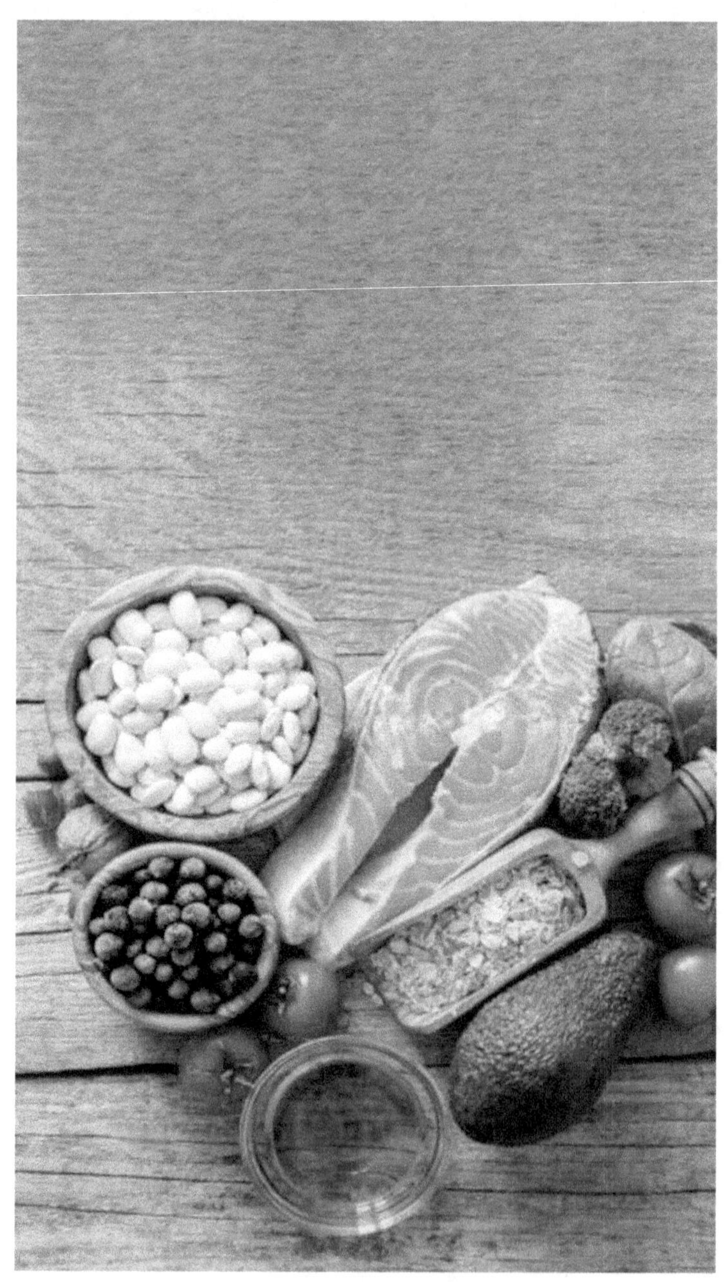

COPYRIGHT

TABLE OF CONTENTS

Table of Contents

INTRODUCTION

FATTY LIVER

Fatty liver disease develops when fat accumulates in liver cells, leading to inflammation and potential liver damage. This condition is commonly associated with factors such as obesity, diabetes, hypertension, and elevated cholesterol levels. It can be classified into two primary types:

Non-alcoholic Fatty Liver Disease (NAFLD): This variant affects individuals who consume minimal or no alcohol and is prevalent in developed nations. NAFLD is frequently correlated with obesity and metabolic syndrome.

Alcoholic Fatty Liver Disease (AFLD): AFLD emerges from excessive alcohol consumption and represents the initial stage of alcohol-induced liver disease.

While symptoms of fatty liver disease might not manifest in the early stages, as the condition progresses, individuals may experience fatigue, weakness, weight loss, abdominal discomfort, jaundice, and swelling in the abdominal region and extremities.

To manage fatty liver disease effectively, the following general recommendations are advised:

Adhere to a Balanced Diet: Prioritize a diet abundant in fruits, vegetables, whole grains, and lean proteins, while limiting saturated fats, trans fats, refined carbohydrates, and added sugars. Reducing consumption of processed foods and sugary beverages is also recommended.

Maintain a Healthy Weight: Implement a regimen comprising both dietary modifications and regular physical activity to achieve and sustain a healthy weight. Even modest weight loss can mitigate fat accumulation in the liver.

Engage in Regular Exercise: Participate in consistent physical activity such as walking, jogging, swimming, or cycling for at least 30 minutes most days of the week. Exercise aids in enhancing insulin sensitivity, diminishing liver fat, and bolstering overall well-being.

Restrict Alcohol Intake: For individuals afflicted with alcoholic fatty liver disease, minimizing or abstaining from alcohol consumption entirely is imperative, as even moderate intake can exacerbate liver damage.

Address Underlying Medical Conditions: Effectively manage coexisting conditions like diabetes, hypertension, and hypercholesterolemia through appropriate medication, lifestyle adjustments, and routine medical supervision.

Avoid Rapid Weight Loss: Eschew crash diets or rapid weight loss schemes, as they may exacerbate liver inflammation. Opt instead for gradual, sustainable weight reduction achieved through wholesome eating habits and regular exercise.

Monitor Medication Usage: Comply with your healthcare provider's guidance regarding medication and supplement usage, as certain medications may necessitate adjustments or avoidance in individuals with fatty liver disease.

Regular Medical Evaluations: Attend scheduled check-ups with your healthcare provider to monitor liver function, address potential complications, and adapt treatment strategies as warranted.

It is imperative to seek personalized advice and management from a healthcare provider for optimal care of fatty liver disease, as approaches may differ based on individual circumstances and the severity of the condition.

FATTY LIVER DIET

A dietary approach tailored for individuals with fatty liver disease is designed to diminish the accumulation of fat in the liver, foster liver well-being, and address correlated risk factors like obesity, diabetes, and elevated cholesterol levels. Below are some overarching dietary directives for managing fatty liver disease:

Reduce Saturated and Trans Fats: Minimize the intake of foods abundant in saturated and trans fats, including red meat, processed meats, full-fat dairy products, fried items, and commercially baked goods.

Opt for Healthy Fats: Select sources of healthy fats such as olive oil, avocado, nuts, seeds, and fatty fish like salmon and mackerel. These fats are rich in omega-3 fatty acids, renowned for their anti-inflammatory properties, potentially benefiting liver health.

Augment Fiber Consumption: Integrate a wealth of high-fiber foods into your diet, such as fruits, vegetables, whole grains, legumes, and nuts. Fiber aids in digestion, regulates blood sugar levels, and may assist in weight management.

Emphasize Lean Proteins: Include lean protein sources in your meals, such as poultry, fish, tofu, beans, lentils, and low-fat dairy products. These proteins offer essential nutrients without contributing excess saturated fat to your dietary intake.

Curtail Added Sugars and Refined Carbohydrates: Limit the consumption of sugary foods and beverages, along with refined carbohydrates like white bread, white rice, and sugary cereals. These items can foster weight gain and exacerbate insulin resistance, both of which are risk factors for fatty liver disease.

Monitor Portion Sizes: Be vigilant about portion sizes to avoid overeating, as surplus calorie intake can lead to weight gain and the accumulation of fat in the liver. Utilize smaller plates and practice mindful eating to manage portion sizes effectively.

Maintain Adequate Hydration: Ensure adequate water intake throughout the day to support liver function. Restrict the consumption of sugary drinks and alcohol, as they can contribute to liver damage and weight gain.

Limit Alcohol Intake: If you suffer from alcoholic fatty liver disease, it is imperative to abstain from alcohol entirely or moderate your consumption as advised by your healthcare provider. Alcohol can exacerbate liver damage and impede treatment endeavors.

Moderate Sodium Consumption: Scale back on sodium intake by curtailing processed and packaged foods, as well as salty snacks and condiments. Excessive sodium consumption can foster fluid retention and potentially exacerbate liver inflammation.

Seek Expert Guidance: Consult with a registered dietitian or healthcare professional to receive tailored dietary recommendations aligned with your individual needs and medical history. They can assist you in crafting a well-rounded meal plan conducive to liver health and overall well-being.

By adhering to these dietary guidelines and adopting healthy lifestyle habits, individuals with fatty liver disease can enhance liver function, mitigate associated risk factors, and cultivate long-term health prospects.

BENEFITS OF DIET FOR FATTY LIVER DISEASE

A dietary strategy customized for fatty liver disease confers multiple advantages aimed at enhancing liver health, managing associated risk factors, and fostering overall well-being. Here are the primary benefits of adhering to a diet specifically crafted for fatty liver:

Reduction of Liver Fat Accumulation: A diet oriented toward fatty liver disease targets the reduction of fat buildup within the liver, crucial for enhancing liver function and thwarting further liver deterioration.

Enhanced Liver Function: By furnishing vital nutrients and bolstering metabolic processes, a nourishing diet can elevate liver function and facilitate the revitalization of liver cells, culminating in improved overall liver health.

Weight Regulation: Many dietary approaches for fatty liver disease prioritize weight loss or weight control, recognizing obesity as a prominent risk factor for the condition. By attaining and sustaining a healthy weight, individuals can mitigate liver fat accumulation and enhance liver health.

Management of Metabolic Risk Factors: Dietary interventions for fatty liver disease commonly address underlying metabolic risk factors such as obesity, insulin resistance, diabetes, and elevated cholesterol levels. By fostering better regulation of blood sugar, lipid profile, and overall metabolic health, a wholesome diet can curtail the likelihood of complications associated with these conditions.

Reduction of Inflammation: Certain dietary constituents, including antioxidants, omega-3 fatty acids, and anti-inflammatory foods, exhibit the capacity to diminish inflammation in the liver and across the body. Through inflammation reduction, a nutritious diet can assuage symptoms and impede the advancement of fatty liver disease.

Prevention of Liver Damage: A diet abundant in nutrients and low in detrimental substances (e.g., alcohol and processed foods) can forestall further liver damage and the onset of complications linked to fatty liver disease, encompassing conditions like liver fibrosis, cirrhosis, and liver cancer.

Facilitation of Liver Detoxification: Certain foods and nutrients can aid the liver's intrinsic detoxification processes, facilitating the elimination of toxins and waste substances from the body. By integrating these foods into the diet, individuals can bolster liver health and functionality.

Promotion of Overall Well-being: In addition to fortifying liver health, a wholesome diet for fatty liver disease can bolster overall well-being by furnishing essential nutrients, sustaining energy levels, and reducing the risk of other chronic ailments.

Improved Quality of Life: Through symptom alleviation, complication risk reduction, and the promotion of superior overall health, a diet tailored for fatty liver disease can heighten the quality of life for individuals grappling with the condition.

Long-term Health Benefits: Embracing a nutritious diet for fatty liver disease can yield enduring health dividends beyond liver health, encompassing diminished susceptibility to cardiovascular disease, diabetes, and other obesity-related maladies.

In sum, adhering to a diet calibrated for fatty liver disease confers myriad benefits spanning liver health, metabolic well-being, and overall vitality. Collaborating with a healthcare provider or registered dietitian to devise a personalized dietary blueprint tailored to individual requisites and medical history is imperative.

EXERCISE AND LIVER

The relationship between the liver and exercise is multifaceted, with physical activity playing a significant role in promoting liver health and overall well-being. Here's an exploration of how exercise impacts the liver:

Reduction of Liver Fat: Regular exercise has been shown to reduce liver fat accumulation, particularly in individuals with non-alcoholic fatty liver disease (NAFLD). Physical activity helps mobilize stored fat for energy expenditure, thereby decreasing fat deposition in the liver and improving liver function.

Improvement in Insulin Sensitivity: Exercise enhances insulin sensitivity, which is beneficial for individuals with insulin resistance, a common feature of NAFLD and type 2 diabetes. By improving insulin sensitivity, exercise helps regulate blood sugar levels and reduces the risk of metabolic complications associated with liver disease.

Promotion of Weight Loss: Exercise is a cornerstone of weight management and plays a crucial role in achieving and maintaining a healthy weight. Since obesity is a major risk factor for fatty liver disease and other liver conditions, engaging in regular physical activity can contribute to weight loss and reduce the burden on the liver.

Enhanced Metabolic Health: Beyond weight loss, exercise improves overall metabolic health by lowering blood pressure, reducing cholesterol levels, and promoting cardiovascular fitness. These benefits contribute to a healthier metabolic profile, which is essential for liver health and function.

Reduction of Liver Inflammation: Exercise has anti-inflammatory effects throughout the body, including the liver. By reducing systemic inflammation, exercise may help alleviate liver inflammation and prevent the progression of liver disease.

Prevention of Liver Fibrosis: Liver fibrosis, the accumulation of scar tissue in the liver, is a common consequence of chronic liver injury. Research suggests that regular exercise may help prevent or slow the progression of liver fibrosis by promoting liver regeneration and reducing inflammation.

Enhanced Liver Blood Flow: Exercise increases blood flow to the liver, which facilitates the delivery of oxygen and nutrients essential for liver function. Improved blood flow also supports the removal of toxins and waste products from the liver, promoting detoxification and overall liver health.

Reduction of Liver Cancer Risk: Some studies suggest that regular exercise may lower the risk of liver cancer, particularly in individuals with chronic liver disease. Exercise may exert protective effects against liver cancer by reducing liver fat accumulation, inflammation, and oxidative stress.

Improvement in Liver Enzyme Levels: Exercise has been associated with lower levels of liver enzymes, such as alanine aminotransferase (ALT) and aspartate aminotransferase (AST), which are markers of liver health. Lower liver enzyme levels indicate reduced liver inflammation and improved liver function.

Psychological Benefits: In addition to its physiological effects, exercise offers numerous psychological benefits, including stress reduction, improved mood, and enhanced quality of life. These psychological benefits are essential for overall well-being and may indirectly support liver health by reducing stress-related liver damage.

In summary, exercise plays a pivotal role in promoting liver health through various mechanisms, including the reduction of liver fat, improvement in insulin sensitivity, promotion of weight loss, enhancement of metabolic health, reduction of liver inflammation, prevention of liver fibrosis, enhancement of liver blood flow, reduction of liver cancer risk, improvement in liver enzyme levels, and provision of psychological benefits. Integrating regular exercise into one's lifestyle is crucial for maintaining optimal liver function and preventing liver-related complications.

FATTY LIVER DIET RECIPES

Grilled Salmon with Avocado Salsa

Ingredients:

- 4 salmon fillets

- 2 ripe avocados, diced

- 1 small red onion, finely chopped

- 1 tomato, diced

- Fresh cilantro, chopped

- Lime juice

- Salt and pepper to taste

Instructions:

- Preheat the grill to medium-high heat.

- Season the salmon fillets with salt and pepper.

- Grill the salmon for about 4-5 minutes per side until cooked through.

- In a bowl, combine diced avocado, red onion, tomato, cilantro, lime juice, salt, and pepper to make the salsa.

- Serve the grilled salmon topped with avocado salsa.

Baked Lemon Herb Chicken

Ingredients:

- 4 boneless, skinless chicken breasts

- 2 lemons, juiced and zested

- 2 cloves garlic, minced

- 2 tablespoons fresh herbs (such as thyme, rosemary, or parsley), chopped

- 2 tablespoons olive oil

- Salt and pepper to taste

Instructions:

- Preheat the oven to 375°F (190°C).

- In a small bowl, whisk together lemon juice, lemon zest, minced garlic, chopped herbs, olive oil, salt, and pepper.

- Place the chicken breasts in a baking dish and pour the lemon herb mixture over them, ensuring they are evenly coated.

- Bake for 25-30 minutes until the chicken is cooked through and juices run clear.

Zucchini Noodles with Turkey Meatballs

Ingredients:

- 2 large zucchinis, spiralized into noodles

- 1 pound ground turkey

- 1/4 cup breadcrumbs

- 1 egg

- 2 cloves garlic, minced

- 1 teaspoon Italian seasoning

- Salt and pepper to taste

- Olive oil

- Marinara sauce (store-bought or homemade)

Instructions:

- Preheat the oven to 375°F (190°C).

- In a bowl, combine ground turkey, breadcrumbs, egg, minced garlic, Italian seasoning, salt, and pepper. Mix until well combined.

- Shape the mixture into meatballs and place them on a baking sheet lined with parchment paper.

- Bake the meatballs for 20-25 minutes until cooked through.

- In a skillet, heat olive oil over medium heat. Add zucchini noodles and sauté for 2-3 minutes until tender.

- Serve the zucchini noodles topped with marinara sauce and turkey meatballs.

Asian-Style Baked Cod

Ingredients:

- 4 cod fillets

- 2 tablespoons soy sauce (or tamari for gluten-free)

- 1 tablespoon honey

- 1 tablespoon rice vinegar

- 1 tablespoon sesame oil

- 2 cloves garlic, minced

- 1 teaspoon grated ginger

- Sesame seeds and chopped green onions for garnish

Instructions:

- Preheat the oven to 400°F (200°C).

- In a small bowl, whisk together soy sauce, honey, rice vinegar, sesame oil, minced garlic, and grated ginger.

- Place the cod fillets in a baking dish and pour the sauce over them, ensuring they are evenly coated.

- Bake for 12-15 minutes until the fish is cooked through and flakes easily with a fork.

- Garnish with sesame seeds and chopped green onions before serving.

Mediterranean Chickpea Salad

Ingredients:

- 2 cans chickpeas, drained and rinsed

- 1 cucumber, diced

- 1 bell pepper, diced

- 1/2 red onion, thinly sliced

- 1 cup cherry tomatoes, halved

- 1/4 cup Kalamata olives, pitted and sliced

- 1/4 cup crumbled feta cheese

- Fresh parsley, chopped

- Lemon juice

- Olive oil

- Salt and pepper to taste

Instructions:

31

- In a large bowl, combine chickpeas, diced cucumber, diced bell pepper, sliced red onion, halved cherry tomatoes, sliced Kalamata olives, and crumbled feta cheese.

- Drizzle with lemon juice and olive oil, and season with salt and pepper to taste. Toss to combine.

- Sprinkle with chopped fresh parsley before serving.

Tofu and Vegetable Stir-Fry

Ingredients:

- 1 block firm tofu, cubed

- 2 cups mixed vegetables (such as broccoli, bell peppers, carrots, and snap peas)

- 2 cloves garlic, minced

- 1 tablespoon ginger, grated

- 2 tablespoons low-sodium soy sauce (or tamari for gluten-free)

- 1 tablespoon rice vinegar

- 1 tablespoon sesame oil

- Cooked brown rice or quinoa for serving

- Sesame seeds for garnish

Instructions:

- Press the tofu to remove excess moisture, then cut it into cubes.

- In a large skillet or wok, heat sesame oil over medium-high heat. Add minced garlic and grated ginger, and sauté for 1 minute.

- Add cubed tofu to the skillet and cook until lightly browned on all sides.

- Add mixed vegetables to the skillet and stir-fry until tender-crisp.

- In a small bowl, whisk together soy sauce and rice vinegar. Pour the sauce over the tofu and vegetables, and toss to combine.

- Serve the tofu and vegetable stir-fry over cooked brown rice or quinoa, garnished with sesame seeds.

Greek Turkey Burgers

Ingredients:

- 1 pound ground turkey

- 1/4 cup crumbled feta cheese

- 1/4 cup diced red onion

- 1/4 cup chopped fresh parsley

- 2 cloves garlic, minced

- 1 teaspoon dried oregano

- Salt and pepper to taste

- Whole wheat burger buns or lettuce wraps

- Tzatziki sauce for serving

Instructions:

- In a bowl, combine ground turkey, crumbled feta cheese, diced red onion, chopped fresh parsley, minced garlic, dried oregano, salt, and pepper.

- Divide the turkey mixture into equal portions and shape them into burger patties.

- Preheat a grill or grill pan over medium-high heat. Grill the turkey burgers for 5-6 minutes per side until cooked through.

- Serve the turkey burgers on whole wheat burger buns or lettuce wraps, topped with tzatziki sauce.

Eggplant Rollatini

Ingredients:

- 2 medium eggplants, thinly sliced lengthwise

- 2 cups ricotta cheese

- 1/4 cup grated Parmesan cheese

- 1 egg

- 1 cup marinara sauce

- Fresh basil leaves for garnish

- Salt and pepper to taste

Instructions:

- Preheat the oven to 375°F (190°C).

- Place the eggplant slices on a baking sheet lined with parchment paper. Sprinkle them with salt and let them sit for 10-15 minutes to release moisture.

- In a bowl, combine ricotta cheese, grated Parmesan cheese, and egg. Season with salt and pepper.

- Blot the excess moisture from the eggplant slices with paper towels. Spread a spoonful of the ricotta mixture onto each eggplant slice and roll them up.

- Spread a thin layer of marinara sauce on the bottom of a baking dish. Place the eggplant rollatini seam side down in the dish.

- Pour the remaining marinara sauce over the eggplant rollatini.

- Bake for 25-30 minutes until the eggplant is tender and the filling is heated through.

- Garnish with fresh basil leaves before serving.

Salmon and Asparagus Foil Packets

Ingredients:

- 4 salmon fillets

- 1 pound asparagus, trimmed

- 2 tablespoons olive oil

- 2 cloves garlic, minced

- 1 lemon, sliced

- Fresh dill for garnish

- Salt and pepper to taste

Instructions:

- Preheat the oven to 400°F (200°C).

- Place each salmon fillet on a piece of aluminum foil large enough to fold over and seal.

- Arrange the trimmed asparagus around the salmon fillets.

- Drizzle olive oil over the salmon and asparagus. Sprinkle minced garlic over the top.

- Place lemon slices on top of each salmon fillet.

- Season everything with salt and pepper to taste.

- Fold the aluminum foil over the salmon and asparagus to create a packet, sealing tightly.

- Place the foil packets on a baking sheet and bake for 15-20 minutes until the salmon is cooked through and the asparagus is tender.

- Garnish with fresh dill before serving.

Cauliflower Crust Pizza

Ingredients:

- 1 medium head cauliflower, grated

- 1 egg

- 1/4 cup grated Parmesan cheese

- 1/2 teaspoon dried oregano

- 1/2 teaspoon garlic powder

- Salt and pepper to taste

- Pizza sauce

- Your choice of toppings (e.g., vegetables, lean meats, olives)

- Mozzarella cheese (optional)

Instructions:

- Preheat the oven to 400°F (200°C).

- Place the grated cauliflower in a microwave-safe bowl and microwave for 5-6 minutes until tender. Let it cool.

- Place the cooked cauliflower in a clean kitchen towel and squeeze out as much moisture as possible.

- In a bowl, combine the cauliflower with egg, grated Parmesan cheese, dried oregano, garlic powder, salt, and pepper.

- Line a baking sheet with parchment paper and spread the cauliflower mixture into a thin, round crust shape.

- Bake for 20-25 minutes until the crust is golden and crispy.

- Remove from the oven and top with pizza sauce, your choice of toppings, and mozzarella cheese if desired.

- Return to the oven and bake for an additional 10-15 minutes until the cheese is melted and bubbly.

Lentil and Vegetable Soup

Ingredients:

- 1 cup dried lentils, rinsed

- 4 cups vegetable broth

- 1 onion, diced

- 2 carrots, diced

- 2 celery stalks, diced

- 2 cloves garlic, minced

- 1 can diced tomatoes

- 2 cups spinach leaves

- 1 teaspoon dried thyme

- 1 teaspoon dried rosemary

- Salt and pepper to taste

Instructions:

43

- In a large pot, combine the dried lentils, vegetable broth, diced onion, diced carrots, diced celery, minced garlic, diced tomatoes (with juices), dried thyme, and dried rosemary.

- Bring the soup to a boil, then reduce the heat and let it simmer for 25-30 minutes until the lentils and vegetables are tender.

- Stir in the spinach leaves and cook for an additional 5 minutes until wilted.

- Season the soup with salt and pepper to taste before serving.

Baked Eggplant Parmesan

Ingredients:

- 2 medium eggplants, sliced into rounds

- 1 cup whole wheat breadcrumbs

- 1/2 cup grated Parmesan cheese

- 2 eggs, beaten

- 2 cups marinara sauce

- 1 cup shredded mozzarella cheese

- Fresh basil leaves for garnish

- Olive oil

- Salt and pepper to taste

Instructions:

- Preheat the oven to 400°F (200°C).

- Place the beaten eggs in one shallow dish and the whole wheat breadcrumbs mixed with grated Parmesan cheese in another shallow dish.

- Dip each eggplant slice into the beaten eggs, then coat them in the breadcrumb mixture.

- Place the breaded eggplant slices on a baking sheet lined with parchment paper. Drizzle with olive oil and season with salt and pepper.

- Bake for 20-25 minutes until the eggplant is tender and the coating is golden brown.

- In a baking dish, spread a thin layer of marinara sauce. Arrange the baked eggplant slices on top of the sauce.

- Top the eggplant slices with the remaining marinara sauce and shredded mozzarella cheese.

- Bake for an additional 15-20 minutes until the cheese is melted and bubbly.

- Garnish with fresh basil leaves before serving.

Miso-Glazed Cod with Stir-Fried Bok Choy

Ingredients for Cod:

- 4 cod fillets

- 3 tablespoons white miso paste

- 2 tablespoons mirin

- 1 tablespoon soy sauce (or tamari for gluten-free)

- 1 tablespoon honey

- 1 teaspoon grated ginger

- 2 cloves garlic, minced

- Sesame seeds for garnish

Ingredients for Stir-Fried Bok Choy:

- 4 baby bok choy, chopped

- 2 cloves garlic, minced

- 1 tablespoon olive oil

- 1 tablespoon low-sodium soy sauce (or tamari for gluten-free)

- 1 teaspoon sesame oil

Instructions:

- Preheat the oven to 400°F (200°C).

- In a small bowl, whisk together white miso paste, mirin, soy sauce, honey, grated ginger, and minced garlic.

- Place the cod fillets on a baking sheet lined with parchment paper. Brush the miso mixture over the cod.

- Bake for 12-15 minutes until the cod is cooked through and flakes easily with a fork.

- While the cod is baking, heat olive oil in a skillet over medium heat. Add minced garlic and chopped bok choy. Stir-fry for 3-4 minutes until the bok choy is tender-crisp.

- Drizzle with soy sauce and sesame oil, and toss to combine.

- Serve the miso-glazed cod with stir-fried bok choy, garnished with sesame seeds.

Quinoa-Stuffed Acorn Squash

Ingredients:

- 2 acorn squash, halved and seeds removed

- 1 cup quinoa, cooked

- 1/2 cup dried cranberries

- 1/4 cup chopped pecans

- 2 tablespoons maple syrup

- 1 tablespoon olive oil

- 1 teaspoon ground cinnamon

- Salt and pepper to taste

Instructions:

- Preheat the oven to 400°F (200°C).

- Place the acorn squash halves cut side down on a baking

  sheet lined with parchment paper. Bake for 25-30 minutes

  until tender.

- In a bowl, combine cooked quinoa, dried cranberries, chopped pecans, maple syrup, olive oil, ground cinnamon, salt, and pepper.

- Once the squash is tender, flip them over and fill each half with the quinoa stuffing.

- Return the stuffed squash to the oven and bake for an additional 10-15 minutes until heated through.

- Serve hot as a side dish or light meal.

Shrimp and Vegetable Stir-Fry with Cauliflower Rice

Ingredients:

- 1 pound shrimp, peeled and deveined

- 1 head cauliflower, grated into rice-like texture

- 2 cups mixed vegetables (such as bell peppers, snap peas, carrots)

- 2 cloves garlic, minced

- 1 tablespoon grated ginger

- 2 tablespoons low-sodium soy sauce (or tamari for gluten-free)

- 1 tablespoon hoisin sauce

- 1 teaspoon sesame oil

- 2 green onions, chopped

- Sesame seeds for garnish

Instructions:

- In a wok or large skillet, heat sesame oil over medium-high heat. Add minced garlic and grated ginger, and sauté for 1 minute.

- Add mixed vegetables to the skillet and stir-fry until tender-crisp.

- Push the vegetables to one side of the skillet and add the shrimp. Cook for 2-3 minutes until pink and cooked through.

- Stir in the grated cauliflower rice and cook for an additional 2-3 minutes until heated through.

- In a small bowl, whisk together soy sauce and hoisin sauce. Pour the sauce over the shrimp and vegetable mixture, and toss to combine.

- Garnish with chopped green onions and sesame seeds before serving.

Sesame Ginger Tofu Stir-Fry

Ingredients:

- 1 block extra-firm tofu, pressed and cubed

- 2 tablespoons low-sodium soy sauce (or tamari for gluten-free)

- 1 tablespoon sesame oil

- 1 tablespoon rice vinegar

- 1 tablespoon honey

- 1 tablespoon grated ginger

- 2 cloves garlic, minced

- 2 cups mixed vegetables (such as bell peppers, broccoli, snap peas)

- Cooked brown rice for serving

- Sesame seeds and green onions for garnish

Instructions:

- In a bowl, whisk together soy sauce, sesame oil, rice vinegar, honey, grated ginger, and minced garlic to make the sauce.

- Heat a skillet or wok over medium-high heat. Add the cubed tofu and cook until golden brown on all sides.

- Add the mixed vegetables to the skillet and stir-fry for 3-4 minutes until tender-crisp.

- Pour the sauce over the tofu and vegetables, and toss to coat evenly.

- Cook for an additional 2-3 minutes until heated through.

- Serve the sesame ginger tofu stir-fry over cooked brown rice, garnished with sesame seeds and chopped green onions.

Mediterranean Stuffed Bell Peppers

Ingredients:

- 4 bell peppers, halved and seeds removed
- 1 cup cooked quinoa
- 1 can chickpeas, drained and rinsed
- 1/2 cup diced tomatoes
- 1/4 cup chopped Kalamata olives
- 1/4 cup crumbled feta cheese
- 2 tablespoons chopped fresh parsley
- 1 tablespoon olive oil
- 1 teaspoon dried oregano
- Salt and pepper to taste

Instructions:

- Preheat the oven to 375°F (190°C).

- In a bowl, combine cooked quinoa, chickpeas, diced tomatoes, chopped Kalamata olives, crumbled feta cheese, chopped parsley, olive oil, dried oregano, salt, and pepper.

- Spoon the quinoa mixture into the halved bell peppers.

- Place the stuffed peppers in a baking dish and cover with aluminum foil.

- Bake for 25-30 minutes until the peppers are tender.

- Serve hot, garnished with additional fresh parsley if desired.

Salmon Patties with Avocado Sauce

Ingredients for Salmon Patties:

- 2 cans salmon, drained and flaked

- 1/2 cup whole wheat breadcrumbs

- 1/4 cup chopped green onions

- 1 egg, beaten

- 1 tablespoon Dijon mustard

- 1 tablespoon lemon juice

- 1 teaspoon Old Bay seasoning

- Olive oil for cooking

Ingredients for Avocado Sauce:

- 1 ripe avocado

- 1/4 cup Greek yogurt

- 1 clove garlic, minced

- 1 tablespoon lime juice

- Salt and pepper to taste

Instructions:

- In a bowl, combine drained and flaked salmon, whole wheat breadcrumbs, chopped green onions, beaten egg, Dijon mustard, lemon juice, and Old Bay seasoning.

- Form the mixture into patties.

- Heat olive oil in a skillet over medium heat. Cook the salmon patties for 3-4 minutes per side until golden brown and cooked through.

- Meanwhile, prepare the avocado sauce by mashing the ripe avocado in a bowl. Stir in Greek yogurt, minced garlic, lime juice, salt, and pepper.

- Serve the salmon patties with the avocado sauce on top.

Stuffed Portobello Mushrooms with Spinach and Ricotta

Ingredients:

- 4 large Portobello mushrooms, stems removed

- 2 cups fresh spinach, chopped

- 1 cup ricotta cheese

- 1/4 cup grated Parmesan cheese

- 2 cloves garlic, minced

- 1 tablespoon olive oil

- Salt and pepper to taste

- Fresh parsley for garnish

Instructions:

- Preheat the oven to 375°F (190°C).

- Place the Portobello mushrooms on a baking sheet lined with parchment paper.

- In a skillet, heat olive oil over medium heat. Add minced garlic and chopped spinach, and sauté until the spinach is wilted.

- In a bowl, combine sautéed spinach, ricotta cheese, grated Parmesan cheese, salt, and pepper.

- Spoon the spinach and ricotta mixture into the Portobello mushrooms.

- Bake for 20-25 minutes until the mushrooms are tender and the filling is heated through.

- Garnish with fresh parsley before serving.

Cauliflower "Mac" and Cheese

Ingredients:

- 1 medium head cauliflower, cut into florets

- 1 cup low-fat milk

- 1 cup shredded sharp cheddar cheese

- 2 tablespoons cream cheese

- 1/2 teaspoon garlic powder

- Salt and pepper to taste

Instructions:

- Steam the cauliflower florets until tender.

- In a saucepan, heat the milk over medium heat. Stir in the cheddar cheese, cream cheese, garlic powder, salt, and pepper until melted and smooth.

- Add the steamed cauliflower to the cheese sauce and toss to coat.

- Serve as a healthier alternative to macaroni and cheese.

Spaghetti Squash with Turkey Bolognese

62

Ingredients:

- 1 medium spaghetti squash

- 1 pound ground turkey

- 1 onion, diced

- 2 cloves garlic, minced

- 1 can diced tomatoes

- 1 tablespoon tomato paste

- 1 teaspoon dried oregano

- 1 teaspoon dried basil

- Salt and pepper to taste

Instructions:

- Preheat the oven to 400°F (200°C).

- Cut the spaghetti squash in half lengthwise and scoop out the seeds. Place the squash halves cut-side down on a baking sheet.

- Bake for 30-40 minutes until the squash is tender. Use a fork to scrape the flesh into spaghetti-like strands.

- In a skillet, cook the ground turkey, onion, and garlic until the turkey is browned and the onion is soft.

- Stir in the diced tomatoes, tomato paste, dried oregano, dried basil, salt, and pepper. Simmer for 10-15 minutes.

- Serve the turkey bolognese over the spaghetti squash strands.

Thai-Inspired Quinoa Salad

Ingredients:

- 1 cup quinoa, cooked

- 1 cup shredded red cabbage

- 1 carrot, grated

- 1 bell pepper, thinly sliced

- 1/4 cup chopped cilantro

- 1/4 cup chopped mint

- 1/4 cup chopped peanuts

- 2 tablespoons soy sauce

- 1 tablespoon sesame oil

- 1 tablespoon rice vinegar

- 1 tablespoon honey

- 1 teaspoon grated ginger

- Juice of 1 lime

Instructions:

- In a large bowl, combine the cooked quinoa, shredded red cabbage, grated carrot, sliced bell pepper, chopped cilantro, chopped mint, and chopped peanuts.

- In a small bowl, whisk together the soy sauce, sesame oil, rice vinegar, honey, grated ginger, and lime juice.

- Pour the dressing over the quinoa salad and toss to coat.

- Serve chilled or at room temperature.

Egg Roll in a Bowl

Ingredients:

- 1 pound ground turkey or chicken

- 1 onion, diced

- 3 cloves garlic, minced

- 1 tablespoon grated ginger

- 1/4 cup soy sauce

- 1 tablespoon sesame oil

- 1 tablespoon rice vinegar

- 1 teaspoon sriracha sauce (optional)

- 1 head cabbage, thinly sliced

- 2 carrots, julienned

- 4 green onions, chopped

- Sesame seeds for garnish

Instructions:

- In a large skillet, cook the ground turkey or chicken over medium heat until browned.

- Add the diced onion, minced garlic, and grated ginger to the skillet and cook until fragrant.

- Stir in the soy sauce, sesame oil, rice vinegar, and sriracha sauce (if using).

- Add the sliced cabbage and julienned carrots to the skillet. Cook until the cabbage is wilted and the carrots are tender.

- Stir in the chopped green onions.

- Serve the egg roll mixture topped with sesame seeds.

Quinoa Stuffed Bell Peppers

Ingredients:

- 4 large bell peppers

- 1 cup quinoa, cooked

- 1 can black beans, drained and rinsed

- 1 cup corn kernels

- 1 tomato, diced

- 1/2 cup shredded cheddar cheese

- Fresh cilantro, chopped

- Salt and pepper to taste

Instructions:

- Preheat the oven to 375°F (190°C).

- Cut the tops off the bell peppers and remove the seeds and membranes.

- In a bowl, mix cooked quinoa, black beans, corn, diced tomato, shredded cheese, cilantro, salt, and pepper.

- Stuff the bell peppers with the quinoa mixture.

- Place the stuffed peppers in a baking dish and bake for 25-30 minutes until the peppers are tender and the filling is heated through.

Zucchini Noodles with Pesto and Cherry Tomatoes

Ingredients:

- 4 medium zucchinis, spiralized into noodles

- 1 cup cherry tomatoes, halved

- 1/4 cup basil pesto

- 2 tablespoons grated Parmesan cheese (optional)

- Salt and pepper to taste

Instructions:

- Heat a skillet over medium heat and add the spiralized zucchini noodles.

- Cook for 2-3 minutes until the noodles are just tender.

- Add the cherry tomatoes to the skillet and cook for another 1-2 minutes until heated through.

- Remove the skillet from the heat and toss the zucchini noodles and cherry tomatoes with basil pesto.

- Sprinkle with grated Parmesan cheese if desired, and season with salt and pepper.

Greek Yogurt Chicken Salad Lettuce Wraps

Ingredients:

- 2 cups cooked chicken breast, shredded

- 1/2 cup Greek yogurt

- 1/4 cup diced celery

- 1/4 cup diced red onion

- 1/4 cup halved grapes

- 2 tablespoons chopped walnuts

- 1 tablespoon lemon juice

- Salt and pepper to taste

- Lettuce leaves for wrapping

Instructions:

- In a large bowl, combine the shredded chicken breast, Greek yogurt, diced celery, diced red onion, halved grapes, chopped walnuts, and lemon juice.

- Mix until well combined, and season with salt and pepper
  to taste.

- Spoon the chicken salad onto lettuce leaves, and wrap to
  form lettuce wraps.

- Serve chilled.

Quinoa-Stuffed Bell Peppers with Black Beans

Ingredients:

- 4 large bell peppers, halved and seeds removed

- 1 cup cooked quinoa

- 1 can black beans, drained and rinsed

- 1 cup diced tomatoes

- 1/2 cup corn kernels

- 1/4 cup chopped cilantro

- 1 teaspoon ground cumin

- 1/2 teaspoon chili powder

- Salt and pepper to taste

- Shredded cheese for topping (optional)

Instructions:

- Preheat the oven to 375°F (190°C).

- In a large bowl, combine the cooked quinoa, black beans, diced tomatoes, corn kernels, chopped cilantro, ground cumin, chili powder, salt, and pepper.

- Spoon the quinoa mixture into the halved bell peppers.

- Place the stuffed bell peppers in a baking dish, and cover with aluminum foil.

- Bake for 25-30 minutes until the peppers are tender.

- Remove the foil, sprinkle with shredded cheese if desired, and bake for an additional 5 minutes until the cheese is melted.

- Serve hot.

Stuffed Cabbage Rolls

Ingredients:

- 1 head cabbage

- 1 pound lean ground beef or turkey

- 1 cup cooked quinoa

- 1 onion, diced

- 2 cloves garlic, minced

- 1 can diced tomatoes

- 1 tablespoon tomato paste

- 1 teaspoon paprika

- 1/2 teaspoon dried thyme

- Salt and pepper to taste

- Chopped fresh parsley for garnish

Instructions:

- Preheat the oven to 375°F (190°C).

- Bring a large pot of water to a boil. Carefully remove the cabbage leaves, and blanch them in the boiling water for 2-3 minutes until softened. Drain and set aside.

- In a skillet, cook the ground beef or turkey over medium heat until browned. Add the diced onion and minced garlic, and cook until softened.

- Stir in the cooked quinoa, diced tomatoes, tomato paste, paprika, dried thyme, salt, and pepper.

- Place a spoonful of the meat and quinoa mixture onto each cabbage leaf, and roll up tightly.

- Place the stuffed cabbage rolls in a baking dish, seam side down.

- Cover the baking dish with aluminum foil, and bake for 25-30 minutes until heated through.

- Garnish with chopped fresh parsley before serving.

Butternut Squash and Lentil Curry

Ingredients:

- 2 cups diced butternut squash

- 1 cup dried green lentils

- 1 onion, diced

- 2 cloves garlic, minced

- 1 tablespoon grated ginger

- 1 can coconut milk

- 1 can diced tomatoes

- 2 tablespoons curry powder

- 1 teaspoon ground turmeric

- 1 teaspoon ground cumin

- Salt and pepper to taste

- Fresh cilantro for garnish

Instructions:

- In a large pot, combine the diced butternut squash, dried green lentils, diced onion, minced garlic, grated ginger, coconut milk, diced tomatoes, curry powder, ground turmeric, ground cumin, salt, and pepper.

- Bring the mixture to a boil, then reduce the heat and let it simmer for 25-30 minutes until the butternut squash and lentils are tender.

- Adjust the seasoning with salt and pepper if needed.

- Serve the curry hot, garnished with fresh cilantro.

Baked Turkey Meatballs with Zucchini Noodles

Ingredients for Turkey Meatballs:

- 1 pound lean ground turkey

- 1/4 cup whole wheat breadcrumbs

- 1/4 cup grated Parmesan cheese

- 1 egg

- 2 cloves garlic, minced

- 2 tablespoons chopped fresh parsley

- 1 teaspoon dried oregano

- Salt and pepper to taste

Ingredients for Zucchini Noodles:

- 4 medium zucchinis, spiralized into noodles

- 1 tablespoon olive oil

- 2 cloves garlic, minced

- 1/4 teaspoon crushed red pepper flakes

- Salt and pepper to taste

- Chopped fresh basil for garnish

Instructions:

- Preheat the oven to 400°F (200°C). Line a baking sheet with parchment paper.

- In a large bowl, combine the ground turkey, whole wheat breadcrumbs, grated Parmesan cheese, egg, minced garlic, chopped fresh parsley, dried oregano, salt, and pepper. Mix until well combined.

- Roll the turkey mixture into meatballs and place them on the prepared baking sheet.

- Bake for 20-25 minutes until the meatballs are cooked through and browned.

- While the meatballs are baking, heat olive oil in a large skillet over medium heat. Add the minced garlic and

crushed red pepper flakes, and cook for 1-2 minutes until
fragrant.

- Add the spiralized zucchini noodles to the skillet and sauté
for 2-3 minutes until just tender.

- Season the zucchini noodles with salt and pepper to taste.

- Serve the baked turkey meatballs over the zucchini
noodles, garnished with chopped fresh basil.

THANKS   FOR

READING

THIS BOOK.

www.ingramcontent.com/pod-product-compliance
Lightning Source LLC
Chambersburg PA
CBHW050827250726
48653CB00006B/2459